Fabio Correia Lima Nepomuceno
Rosa Camila Gomes Paiva
Walyson Felix da Silva

Blood Vascular Restriction Method in Chondropathy

AF394865

Fabio Correia Lima Nepomuceno
Rosa Camila Gomes Paiva
Walyson Felix da Silva

Blood Vascular Restriction Method in Chondropathy

Physiotherapy for strength gain and muscle hypertrophy in a woman with chondromalacia patellae

ScienciaScripts

Imprint

Any brand names and product names mentioned in this book are subject to trademark, brand or patent protection and are trademarks or registered trademarks of their respective holders. The use of brand names, product names, common names, trade names, product descriptions etc. even without a particular marking in this work is in no way to be construed to mean that such names may be regarded as unrestricted in respect of trademark and brand protection legislation and could thus be used by anyone.

Cover image: www.ingimage.com

This book is a translation from the original published under ISBN 978-613-9-79906-0.

Publisher:
Sciencia Scripts
is a trademark of
Dodo Books Indian Ocean Ltd. and OmniScriptum S.R.L publishing group

120 High Road, East Finchley, London, N2 9ED, United Kingdom
Str. Armeneasca 28/1, office 1, Chisinau MD-2012, Republic of Moldova, Europe
Printed at: see last page
ISBN: 978-620-6-36792-5

FABIO CORREIA LIMA NEPOMUCENO
ROSA CAMILA GOMES PAIVA
WALYSON FELIX DA SILVA

PHYSIOTHERAPEUTIC TREATMENT USING THE
BLOOD VASCULAR RESTRICTION METHOD
TO GAIN STRENGTH AND
MUSCLE HYPERTROPHY IN WOMEN WITH CHONDROPATHY

JOÃO PESSOA
PB

1

I dedicate this, and all my other achievements, first of
all to JEHOVAH GOD and all my family and friends,
for always cheering for me and always supporting me

ACKNOWLEDGMENTS

I thank God first for providing this whole journey and struggle, and showing how important it is to run after our dreams and finally be able to realize it with great success, I thank mine for helping me on this long journey by financing my studies and always encouraging me to do my best, I love you very much.

I thank my internship group for providing great moments together, new knowledge shared with great dedication, I thank the teachers for always being willing to teach and be patient with all students. I thank all my class, because you can be sure that I will miss you all very much. I wish you all success!

I thank everyone for always supporting me and encouraging me to do what I love most, which is being a Physiotherapist.

SUMMARY

The strength training and hypertrophy using the method of RFS (Restriction Blood Flow), has shown through experiments very effective and has been gaining space every day, because showing to be a very beneficial way to gain strength and hypertrophy using low pounds. Some researchers like Nakajima et al. (2006) used the kaatsu Training or RFS in Japan and found good results in gyms, orthopedic clinics and hospitals, in Japan is already widely used such a method, where in 84% of the places surveyed are used these methods kaatsu. Chondropathy refers to diseased cartilage. This condition usually causes pain in the front of the knee and clicking, especially when the person squats, runs, gets up from a chair or goes up and down stairs. The more specific term for this condition is patellofemoral syndrome. Patellar chondropathy presents different stages, depending on the degree of cartilage degeneration: softening, fragmentation or cracks, up to erosion or total loss. This is why it is necessary to consult a doctor immediately, even at the beginning of the pain. If physical activity is insisted upon, cracks in the cartilage can expose the bones to friction, considerably increasing the pain and causing swelling in the affected knee. This is an interventional clinical research with the character of experimental research case study with quantitative approach. The patient involved in the study, diagnosed with patellar chondropathy. The research was carried out at the G+ Academy located on Tancredo Neves Avenue, Mandacaru neighborhood, next to the Madacaruense company; Joao Pessoa PB. An evaluation form created by the researchers and instruments such as the gym machines and sphygmomanometer were used as instruments. The study was approved by the Collegiate of the Physiotherapy Course and, after approval by the Ethics and Research Committee and signing of the informed consent form and letter of consent, data collection was carried out.

Key words: vascular occlusion, chondropathy, physiotherapy

TABLE OF CONTENTS

INTRODUCTION

The reduction of muscle blood flow during resistance exercise has been shown to be very beneficial for gaining muscle mass and strength, such strength and hypertrophy similar to that of high intensity resistance exercise, but using lower intensity during exercise. (LOENNEKE et al., 2010) (LOENNEKE et al., 2012).

We know that blood flow is a very important factor during resistance exercise, as it is the component of oxygen transport to the muscles. Blood flow supplies sufficient oxygen demand and removes by-products from the muscles (ABE et al, 2009).

Hâ about a decade Japanese researchers developed a technique that combined with the strength training (TF) of low intensity (20-50% of 1RM), with blood vascular restriction also well known as KAATSU training (training with vascular occlusion), studies have shown that this method has a very significant result on high intensity strength training (60-80% of 1 RM). (TAKARADA, et al. 2000)

According to Wernbom et al. (2008) when it is prescribed exercises with resistance, the training intensity or load used is considered the most important variable. The intensity of resistance training is often quantified as a function of the maximum weight that can be lifted in a single time, called maximum repetition (1 RM). They believe that the load should be at least 60% of 1 RM in order to stimulate increased strength. For muscle hypertrophy, loads of 6-12 RM are generally recommended, which correspond to 70-80% of 1 RM. However, in a clinical setting it is contraindicated to use maximal load for rehabilitation after any sports injury.

It is believed that blood flow restriction during low-intensity exercise increases muscle endurance, phosphorylation and protein synthesis, and promotes strength gains as much as conventional resistance exercise with high loads. However, the cellular mechanism responsible for the strength gain and hypertrophy induced by blood flow restriction (BFR) are not yet fully known, it is suggested that vascular occlusion causes a stimulation of local metabolism, which in turn stimulates growth factors, primary recruitment of fast twitch fibers and increased protein synthesis (ABE et al, 2014).

Studies show that RFS helps in increasing muscle volume and consequently increasing strength when compared to high intensity exercise, so this study is unanimous, as studies do not prove that blood vascular occlusion has significant negative differences on high intensity training for strength gain and hypertrophy. (KARABULUT et al. 2011)

However, the strong mechanical stress of high-intensity exercises is strongly associated with musculoskeletal injuries, especially in older or elderly people, whose musculoskeletal system is more debilitated. In this context, the Kaatsu Training method emerged. Basically it consists of the use of cuffs to control the pressure exerted on specific points of the body to block the flow of blood to the exercised regions, which consists of a low-intensity resistance training, aiming at reducing venous return causing the accumulation of blood in the blood vessels to induce muscle hypertrophy. This method has been much discussed, because, while some authors report its benefits, showing favorable to its application, others refer to the adverse effects and risks, being totally contrary. Because of this, it is essential to evaluate the data in the literature and the possible physiological changes resulting from the use of the Kaatsu method (ABE et al, 2009).

Nakajima et al. (2006) analyzed the use of Kaatsu in Japan and found good adherence by gyms, hospitals and orthopedic clinics, in which 84% of them had started using it in the last five years. The use of the low-intensity vascular occlusion training method appears to be safe when performed in the pressure range between 50 and 200 mmHg. The same authors report that hemodynamic responses during resistance exercise, even if performed at low intensity, result in increased heart rate, systolic blood pressure, systolic volume and cardiac output. In addition, when high loads are used, diastolic blood pressure also increases.

Nagashima and Inoue (2012) state that the protocol of exercises focused on strengthening the quadriceps is efficient and has benefits, because it is promoted a patellar alignment with the balance of the stabilizing muscles of the patella.

Deliberato (2007), says that the strengthening should be focused on quadriceps, with emphasis on vast medial because it occurs the normality of patellar mobility and control of the entire lower joint and increased flexibility in General. Therefore, for Domingues (2008), muscle strengthening, especially the quadriceps muscles have an active role in reducing the impact, directly influencing the alignment of the patella.

According to Oliveira and Guimaraes (2012), functional bandage or Kinesio Taping (KT) favors pain relief and improved stability, promoting constant mobility without loss of muscle function of the individual, in order to promote sensorio motor stimulation. The objectives of the application of the tape are based on two essential points: 1) the correction of the patella within the femoral trochlea, promoting an increase in contact areas and decreasing joint stress, resulting in a decrease in pain intensity and 2) facilitate the activity (intensity and recruitment) of the vastus internus oblique. (JARDIM, 2009).

The physiotherapeutic methods applied, aim to mitigate the trauma caused by patellofemoral instability and patellar dislocation, reintegrating the muscles, seeking a greater degree of independence, in order to avoid new injuries and provide the patient a gradual and permanent return to their normal life activities (NAGASHIMA; INOUE, 2012).

According to Poton and Polito (2014), the cardiovascular response with resistance exercises with RFS, where systolic and diastolic blood pressure and heart rate are very related. Something that worried other researchers who practiced this training methodology, according to the research they did could be observed that the cardiovascular response related to blood pressure only came to be worrying after the third series of exercise performed with RFS in the upper limbs, in elbow flexion, with 200mmHg throughout the exercise section doing 3 sets of 15 repetitions with 20% of 1RM.

The knee is a joint of great performance, and its structures are fundamental to the development of biomechanics. According to Pardine (2002), the knee provides a good degree of stability performing important function in its extension and flexion movements.

Being a complex joint, the knee is formed by osseous structures, soft tissues, ligaments, tendons and menisci. Anatomically it is composed of femur, patella, fibula, tibia and mainly by the quadriceps muscles (vastus lateralis, vastus medialis, vastus intermedius and rectus femoris), tensor fascia lata, sartorius, grâcil, located posteriorly, the ischio-tibial muscles (semimembranâceus, semitendinosus and biceps femoris), popliteus and gastrocnemius. The ligaments and menisci are respectively: anterior cruciate ligament (ACL), posterior cruciate ligament (PCL), tibial collateral ligament, fibular collateral ligament and patellar ligament, as for the menisci, medial and lateral meniscus. Finally, their joints are called femoropatellar, meniscofemoral, meniscofibular and tibiofibular (NETTER, 2000; PUTZ; PABST, 2000).

The articular system has the function of connecting different bones of the human body, and are classified based on their anatomical characteristics or the type of movement they perform. Structurally designated in fibrous joints (Sinartrose), cartilaginous (Amphiarthrosis) and synovial (Diarthrosis) subdivided into monoaxial, biaxial and triaxial (TORTOTA; DERRICKSON, 2012). Femoropatellar joint located between the patella and the osseous structures and soft tissues (LIMA; MEJIA, 2016).

The sum of the forces between the vastus intermedius and the vastus lateralis causes a tendency for lateral displacement of the patella. The medial force is represented by the sum of the forces of the vastus medialis longus and the vastus medialis oblique. When the forces of the vastus medialis oblique and the vastus lateralis are balanced, the resultant of these forces is directed towards the upper thigh. But if there is no such balance, changes occur in the positioning of the patella. It is more common to find the vast medial weaker in relation to the lateral, given that it is the largest and strongest muscle of the quadriceps femoris; In addition, the vast medial oblique has its oblique fibers, making it difficult to gain strength and hypertrophy in relation to the vast lateral (MONNERAT, 2010).

A study by Monnerat (2010), observed that after anterior cruciate ligament injury, the vastus lateralis showed loss of muscle mass at about 8 weeks after injury, while the vastus medialis showed reduction after 4 weeks.

It was also found that in humans there is a large reduction in the muscle mass of the oblique medial vastus in relation to the lateral vastus in individuals with patellar dislocation. These studies show that biomechanical changes, such as some knee injuries, can influence muscle imbalance and, if not treated correctly, lead the person to develop patellar chondromalacia (MONNERAT, 2010).

Chondropathy refers to diseased cartilage. This condition usually causes pain in the front of the knee and clicking, especially when the person squats, runs, gets up from a chair or goes up and down stairs. The more specific term for this condition is patellofemoral syndrome. The highest incidences in women in relation to the Q angle, which is the relationship between the knee hip between the knee patella and lateral part of the antero superior iliac hip, the misalignment of this angle leads the knees to be inward in valgus in this way the patella is more lateralized promoting greater wear of the cartilage during movement, very common in women because of having the hip be wider because of genetic characteristics due to pregnancy the relationship and also little strength in the knee stabilizing muscles such as iliotibial tract, quadriceps (BRUKNER et al. 2006).

Women also often use heels and this increases patellar pressure when walking and promoting greater wear, in athletes there is also a high incidence due to excessive exercise and mainly due to exercise failure and recovery failure. A lower activation of quadriceps and greater activation of tlbias so occurring patellar pain and also some studies show that the shortening of the quadriceps also influence the increase in patellar pressure. The chondropathy also known as runner's knee and patellofemoral syndrome, refers to the early stages of patellar concromalacia, is a chronic degenerative pathology of the posterior surface cartilage of the patella generating discomfort and pain in the lateral and posterior part of the patella. The causes of chondropathies are still many relative as already mentioned above also has a relationship not only by muscle weakness but also the shortening of some muscle groups, where they are also related to anatomical factors, physiological and structural factors as one of them women for their genetic factor of having the hip but wide so leading a muscle lack of control and leading the knees to stay inside (valgismo), exerclcios performed incorrectly, overtraining, incorrect and exaggerated angulations, another factor is the traumas that can hinder the inadequate nutrition of the structure in question due to fissures produced. (NAIANE, 2014)

The above-mentioned author says that patellar chondropathy presents different stages, according to the degree of cartilage degeneration: softening, fragmentation or fissures, up to erosion or total loss. This is why it is necessary to consult a doctor immediately, even when the pain starts. If physical activity is insisted upon, cracks in the cartilage can expose the bones to friction, considerably increase the pain and cause swelling in the affected knee. Surgical treatment is the last resort as it will cause limitation of sporting activity.

Sedentary people, the elderly, and patients with some cardiac pathologies, patients with joint injuries, pre-surgical joint injuries, post-surgical joint injuries and others, have training with RFS, a good alternative to bring good results, thus benefiting those who cannot obtain high training intensities.

According to the Brazilian Society of Arthroscopy and Sports Traumatology (2011), dislocation is a serious injury in which there is sudden, partial or total displacement of the patella by local trauma. The anatomical causes are related to alterations of the patella (high) and knee (valgus). According to data collected, when a first dislocation occurs, the individual has approximately 15% chance of getting a new recurrence.

I aroused a divine interest in studying and delving into this subject because knowing its good results, and thinking about future good results with post and pre-surgical patients, such as ACL, chondropathy, or any other knee injury that needs to gain muscle volume, and decrease pain consequently without using too much intensity, and have the need to train and work with low intensity (kilage) and have good results of strength gain and muscle hypertrophy. As well as the high intensity exercise where it is worked over 60 to 80% of 1 RM, to obtain good results, the exercise with RFS brings the benefit of working with only 20 to 50% of 1 RM, to increase the gain of strength and hypertrophy, results similar to high intensity.

According to all the studies cited above, it can be observed that contrary to what is widely known today to have a good gain in muscle mass and strength, it is necessary to practice high intensity exercise with 60-80% of 1RM. The training using the RFS method, showed something totally contrary to the high intensity strength training, only using the restriction of blood flow during exercise using a pressure cuff where it can be used from 50 to 200mmhg, in the most proximal part of the limb to be trained associated with resistance exercise with only 20-50% of 1RM, it is possible to gain a good muscle volume and strength of the trained limb. Is there a decrease in pain using the RFS method to gain strength and hypertrophy in women with chondropathy?

It was believed that training with RFS (blood vascular restriction) would show a good result in people with chondropathy to gain strength and hypertrophy and decrease localized pain, using only 20% to 50% of 1RM, thus avoiding high intensity exercises that have the same objective, using training loads of 60% to 80% of 1RM, as some studies prove, however, the alternative of applying this method, in people who have limitations to practice high intensity exercises. Therefore, the following hypothesis is launched: strength and hypertrophy training using RFS decreased pain and increased strength and muscle volume in women with chondropathy. Strength and hypertrophy training using RFS did not decrease pain and did not increase strength and muscle volume in women with chondropathy.

In view of this problem, the main objective of the research was to carry out a case study on

RFS applied in a woman with chondropathy, through a physiotherapeutic evaluation, reporting its main clinical manifestations of chondropathy and the importance of the physiotherapist using new methods as a treatment of pathology.

The chapters immediately after will bring a good and deep definition of how the training reaction can act on the individual's body. In chapter 1 will report on the vascular occlusion of its definition and how it is performed in training, how it was created and when it was discovered and by whom, also showing several researches carried out with this method for different objectives, its benefits, indications and contraindications.

Chapter 2 describes what patellar chondropathy is, talking a little about what chondropathy really is, its phases and risks. In chapter 3 conceptualize the muscle physiology describing in detail what it is and how it is involved in training, also conceptualizing the energy sources for muscle contraction and describing what is contraction force and muscle hypertrophy.

Chapter 4 presents the methodological route talking a little about the performance of the research as it was performed, where it was performed, objects used to perform the intervention, results and discussion.

CHAPTER 1 - PHYSIOTHERAPY AND BLOOD VASCULAR OCCLUSION OR RESTRICTION (RFS)

Roque et al (2012) describe in their article the conservative method as initial treatment in patellofemoral dysfunctions, aiming to alleviate pain, and recover the function such as total range of motion, through therapeutic modalities such as muscle strengthening and stretching, reducing patellofemoral overload.

Cryotherapy or cold therapy is the application of any substance applied to the body that results in decreased body temperature and tissue (FERREIRA; FERNANDES, 2012; BRANCO et al, 2005). The heat is removed from the body and absorbed by cold and gets local and systemic responses and are correlated with temperature, duration of treatment, and the area subjected to treatment (STARKEY, 2001; FREITAS; LUZARDO, 2013).

According to Carvalho and Chierichetti (2006), cryotherapy is applied to reduce edema, because it has anti-inflammatory and analgesic effect. The action of cold in the immediate treatment in acute injuries, decreases the recovery time and a faster return to functional activities in which it promotes reduction of inflammation, reduction of edema and hematoma, reducing the pain threshold and a faster tissue repair and shorter rehabilitation time.

According to Miyamoto, Soriano and Cabral (2010), patellar misalignment and pain are caused by muscle shortening, and to improve the shortening, passive and active stretching techniques were used for the anterior and posterior chain muscle groups of the lower limbs lasting thirty seconds in all physiotherapy sessions.

For Cabral et al (2007), the stretches have benefits in increasing flexibility and improved functioning and are necessary for prevention and rehabilitation of injuries, the most used are the static stretches applied safely and according to the patient's tolerance. The flexibility exercises in lower limbs assume a significant role to minimize the compressive forces acting on the patella (PECCIN; CHAMLIAN, 2005).

The treatment of patellofemoral instability syndrome is guided to the rehabilitation of quadriceps muscle activity, since it contributes to the improvement of symptoms. Isometric strengthening exercises are performed without the movement of the joint, i.e., there are no changes in muscle length (KISNER; COLBY, 2005).

The exercises of open kinetic chain (CCA) and closed kinetic chain (CCF) according to Noble (2011), points improvement in pain and muscle strength, becoming recommended in therapy. For Prentice (2008), among the exercises of CCF stands out the mini-squat, which comprises sliding against the wall with the aid of a Swiss ball, step climbs and ergonomic bike.

Generally the treatment for chondromalacia is conservative and will not reverse the injury, but there will be improvements in knee function and decreased pain (FULKERSON, 2000). Mello (2006) says that the knee has the function of absorbing and directing force to the lower limb and, therefore, the treatment needs to be functional. Firstly, conventional physiotherapy programs (cryotherapy, etc.) are performed, which are efficient in the edema and severe pain phase. The next step is to improve the function of the knee, which can be achieved by physiotherapy exercises and then muscle strengthening. The big problem is the difficulty that people have in maintaining physical activity throughout their lives, and then they may experience symptoms again.

Mello (2006) states that one of the objectives to improve pain symptoms is to reduce the contact force between the patella and the femur, which varies between open and closed kinetic chain exercises. It is therefore necessary to know this variation for the treatment to be efficient. The open kinetic chain is characterized by exercises aimed at working a particular muscle with the distal segment free. The closed kinetic chain exercise exists when the distal segment is fixed, such as getting up from a chair, going up and down stairs, which in turn becomes more functional for people.

In open kinetic chain exercises, the force is greatest in flexion from 90 degrees to 0 degree in extension, because the center of gravity is in front of the knee and at these angles the contact area between the patella and the femur decreases. Up to 30 degrees the force angle is very small and does not generate high stress on the patellofemoral joint. Therefore, for individuals with chondromalacia, open kinetic chain exercises between 0 and 15 degrees and 50 and 90 degrees should be used. The maximum pressure is around 35 to 45 degrees, where the angle is greater (ANDREWS, 2000).

Haupenthal (2006) states that in the closed kinetic chain exercise, the force increases from 0 to 90 degrees, because the center of gravity is behind the knee. The increase in force is increased according to the contact area up to 60 degrees and, from this angle, the contact area increases greatly, but does not cause damage to healthy knees. In this type of exercise there is co-contraction of the tibial ischium. According to Eisenhart (2004), from the angle of 60 degrees, co-contraction causes the tibia to move posteriorly and rotate to the side, increasing the pressure on the patella. The closed kinetic chain exercises, for those who have this type of injury, should be done until close to 50 degrees, to avoid the changes mentioned. Belleman (2003) says that the knee without injury is adapted to the maximum pressure between the patella and the femur at 90 degrees, because it is from this point that the cartilage is thicker.

Many professionals seek more selective recruitment of the vastus medialis muscle in order to have better success in treatment and there are still controversies regarding the most advantageous exercise to strengthen it in this way. A study by Stoutenberg (2005) investigated the electromyographic variations between the vastus medialis, vastus lateralis and rectus femoris muscles due to the position of the tibia during exercise in the extensor chair and concluded that there are no significant differences in relation to the position of the tibia. Willis (2005) observed that exercise on the bicycle in lateral rotation provides greater activation of the vastus medialis, but the difference between with or without tibial rotation did not cause significant differences. The results of these two studies can be explained by the knee performing lateral rotation only when it is flexed to 90 degrees, thus hindering the more selective recruitment of the vastus medialis.

According to Popelas (2005) for the selective recruitment of the vastus medialis, there are differences between the closed kinetic chain exercises depending on the flexion angle. For closed kinetic chain, the angle should be up to 50 degrees of flexion (in addition to the femoropatellar stress is lower); in open kinetic chain, should be done exercises with angulation from 50 degrees of extension. Bakhtiary (2008) states that exercises in closed kinetic chain are more efficient in the treatment for people with chondromalacia patellae, because they are more functional exercises and easier to use, considering that the femoropatellar stress in open kinetic chain exercises is very large in the "middle" of the movement, requiring another person to help.

The RFS method was developed by a Japanese a few decades ago, in his respective country Japan. It happened respectively in the year 1967, when Sato, the main creator of this training method, kaatsu training, decided to start some experiments applying this method to his own body, based on a personal experience where in a Buddhist temple he knelt on his own legs and felt numbness in both legs. (LENZI, 2016)

Determined to understand this phenomenon that happened to his body, he began a series of experiments, using his own body as an object of study and subjected his limbs to high pressure values such as 600mmhg and above, for a very long time. As he didn't know the specific location for application was subjected to several tests on your own body to know the most correct place to apply and decrease blood flow, in the year 1967, Sato managed to establish an effective and safe method, thus being able to create parameters so that it was possible to determine the appropriate pressure in the training used kaatsu training and counter-resistance training. (LENZI, 2016).

The author also mentions that in 1973, Sato suffered a skiing accident, where he broke some bones and ruptured some ligaments. The perspective he had at that time was muscle atrophy, where until then it was the natural consequence of this type of injury, Sato began to use his training method, kaatsu. Where surprisingly in a short period of time of 2 weeks, the doctor who accompanied him diagnosed that there had been no prevention of muscle atrophy typical of these cases, but on the contrary, the muscles had hypertrophied. Through this event Sato could come to a conclusion, that he had indeed established the basic technique for kaatsu training.

Strength and hypertrophy training using the RFS method has shown through experiments a lot of efficiency and is gaining more space every day, as it proves to be a very beneficial way to gain strength and hypertrophy using low weights. Strength and hypertrophy training today has been increasingly sought after by young people, adults and the elderly, and aiming to gain lean mass and strength, high intensity training is using 60% to 80% of 1RM, with the same objective. The RFS method is used only with 20% to 50% of 1RM, so several evidences show that the RFS method is safe and effective, where they often obtain values equal to or even greater than high intensity training. (TAKARADA, et al., 2000)

Some researchers like Nakajima et al. (2006) used kaatsu in Japan and found good results in gyms, orthopedic clinics and hospitals, in Japan is already widely used such a method, where in 84% of the places surveyed are used these methods kaatsu.

Another very important factor in this training method is the significant increase in GH (human growth hormone) in blood plasma compared to other training methods. The accumulation of metabolites consequently increases the concentration of GH, this increase was verified in other studies after exercise, a study carried out with young people using vascular occlusion proved that after exercise there is a large increase and accumulation of GH in the blood plasma, where also the greater electrical activity in muscle activity thus recruiting more muscle fibers in the execution of the exercise, the authors also concluded that the gradual increase in lactate in the blood plasma during exercise combined also with hypoxia leading to greater recruitment of motor units. Thus recruiting larger amounts of motor units coming to the conclusion that a significant gain not only of strength, but also of muscle hypertrophy. (TAKARADA et al., 2000)

According to Allan and Borba (2013) it was observed in some studies that there is no standardized or protocolized pressure, ranging from 100mmhg and 200mmhg. Other ways used to determine a certain type of pressure was assessing the systolic pressure at rest. And also 50% to 80% of the individual's full vascular pressure. Most of the studies carried out maintained pressure throughout the exercise protocol performed, also including rest intervals.

Other authors did it differently, performed RFS during exercise, with a pressure of 50-100mmhg, using the super series method for agonist and antagonist in elbow flexors and extensors, 3 exercises for extensors and three for flexors, interval between sets of 30 to 60 seconds with the RFS and intervals between the exercises of 5minutes without the RFS, total time of the RFS of 10-15min, the exercises were performed until concentric fatigue in 4 sets for each exercise, so it was observed but a form of training with RFS. (POPE et al., 2013)

CHAPTER 2 - DESCRIBING CHONDROPATHY

Patellar chondromalacia is a lesion in the articular cartilage of the patella due to excessive friction between the patella and the femur (MOREIRA, 2006). This pathology can occur for various reasons, but mainly by poor alignment of the patella, due to the asymmetry of the vastus medialis and vastus lateralis muscles (BUCKWALTER, 2000). Pereira (1996) verified that the femoropatellar pain, affected by chondromalacia, is very frequent (77%) and a good part of the population feels pain in the anterior part of the knee, since it is one of the consequences of this lesion, but not a diagnosis for it, as many people claim.

Chondropathy refers to diseased cartilage. This pathology usually causes pain in the front of the knee and clicking, especially when the person squats, runs, gets up from a chair or goes up and down stairs. The more specific term for this condition is patellofemoral syndrome. The highest incidences in women are in relation to the Q angle, which is the relationship between the patella of the knee and the lateral part of the antero-anterior iliac hip, the misalignment of this angle leads the knees to be inward in valgus, thus the patella is more lateralized promoting greater wear of the cartilage during movement, very common in women due to the hip is wider, for presenting genetic characteristics related to pregnancy and also by little strength in the knee stabilizing muscles such as the iliotibial tract and quadriceps. (BRUKNER et al, 2006)

According to Monnerat (2010), the patella moves constantly in active knee movements, moving in a pattern with a "C" shape between the femoral condyles. The sum of the forces between the vastus medialis and the vastus lateralis causes a resultant directed towards the upper thigh. But if this balance is not achieved, changes occur in the positioning of the patella, and then the patella moves out of its pattern between the condyles ("C" shape) and the cartilage comes into contact with the femur bone, wearing it out. It is therefore necessary to strengthen the muscle that is out of balance in order to improve the dysfunction.

Women also often use heels and this increases patellar pressure when walking promoting the greatest wear, in athletes also there is a high incidence due to excessive exercise and mainly by failure of exercises and failure to recover. There is a lower activation of the quadriceps and greater activation of hamstrings, thus occurring patellar pain. (NAIANE, 2014)

Zachary et al. (2012) chondropathy also known as runner's knee and patellofemoral syndrome, refers to the early stages of patellar concromalacia, is a chronic degenerative pathology of the posterior surface cartilage of the patella generating discomfort and pain in the lateral and posterior part of the patella. The causes of chondropathies are still many relative as already mentioned above also has relationship not only by muscle weakness but also the shortening of some muscle groups, where they are also related to anatomical factors, physiological and structural factors as one of them women for their genetic factor of having the hip but wide thus leading a muscular lack of control and leading the knees to stay inside (valgism), exercises performed incorrectly, overtraining, incorrect and exaggerated angulations, another factor is the traumas that can hinder the inadequate nutrition of the structure in question due to the fissures produced.

Patellar chondromalacia is a lesion in the articular cartilage of the patella due to excessive friction between the patella and the femur (MOREIRA, 2006). The femoropatellar pain happens very often and the cause of this injury may be due to biomechanical changes: increased Q angle; excessive use of the joint; increased patellofemoral pressure; shortening of the tibial ischium muscles; genetic factors such as lateral rotation of the tibia, high patella, length of the ilio tibial band (which is more frequent in women, because they have wider hips in relation to men); muscle imbalance. Many professionals associate patellofemoral pain to diagnose chondromalacia, but Mello (2006) states that the association of these causes is what can lead someone to develop this pathology; therefore, patellofemoral pain is not a diagnosis for chondromalacia, but one of the consequences. The diagnosis should be given mainly through MRI and the main cause is the muscular imbalance between the vast medial and vast lateral (BUCKWALTER, 2000).

Patellar chondropathy presents different stages, depending on the degree of cartilage degeneration: softening, fragmentation or cracks, up to erosion or total loss. This is why it is necessary to consult a doctor immediately, even at the beginning of the pain. If physical activity is insisted upon, cracks in the cartilage can expose the bones to friction, considerably increasing the pain and causing swelling in the affected knee. Surgical treatment is the last resort as it will cause limitation of sporting activity.

CHAPTER 3 - CONCEPTUALIZING BIOMECHANICS AND MUSCLE PHYSIOLOGY

The patellofemoral joint is composed of the patellar face (femur) and the posterior face of the patella, these two bones need to work in perfect harmony so that there is not only a good patellar slip on the femur, but also so that the femoral condyles can roll, slide and rotate on the tibial plateau (WHITING, 2001).

Perfect patellofemoral function will be strongly influenced by the static (non-contractile structures) and dynamic (contractile structures) stabilizers of the joint. The patella constantly moves in active knee movements, moving in a "C" shaped pattern. In the frontal plane in knee extension at 0 degrees it starts supero - lateral, from the first 40 degrees of flexion the patella becomes more inferiorized and medialized. In the sagittal plane the patella undergoes a flexion of 65 to 75 degrees, which occurs after the flexion of the tibia. From 90 degrees of flexion in the frontal plane the patella is not only being medialized but also undergoes lateralization when the knee is hyperflexed. In the transverse plane the tibia appears to exert a strong influence on the degree of tilt, deviation and rotation of the patella. External rotation of the tibia leads to an increase in patellar tilt, deviation and lateral rotation, whereas the opposite is true for internal rotation of the tibia. Axial rotations of the knee are performed either actively or "automatically". Automatic or involuntary rotations are related to flexion and extension movements and occur mainly at the last degrees of extension or at the beginning of flexion. When the knee is extended, it raises the foot for external rotation.

Conversely when the knee is flexed the leg rotates in internal rotation. The contact areas of the patella with the femur will be established according to the angle of knee flexion and the eccentric contraction force of the quadriceps (OLIVEIRA; GUIMARÂES, 2012).

During knee flexion, the quadriceps produces an upward force, while the patellar cleft supports this force in the opposite direction. The resolution of these forces leads to a posterior outcome, which causes increased compression of the patella with the femur. At angles less than 30 degrees, patellofemoral compression decreases. This means a decrease in contact between the two articular surfaces and a decrease in the resulting force vector directed posteriorly. At this angle the patella is supported by a supra-trochlear fat pad. It should be emphasized that the insertion angle of approximately 0 degree creates a stability vector. The tendon parallel to the bone generates a very small power arm, the quadriceps muscle exerts a much greater work to support the leg in extension and favors stabilization and not displacement. Already the tendon perpendicular to the bone favors displacement and not stabilization (MONERRAT et al, 2010).

Mechanisms of injury to this joint include poor patellar alignment, increased quadriceps angle-(q), hyperpronation of the feet or weakness in the vastus medialis oblique muscle

(MACHADO, 2005).

According to Monnerat (2010), the patellofemoral joint consists of the femur and the posterior face of the patella, which is between the femoral condyles. The patella detaches enough in active movements of the knee; the same and the condyles of the femur are incongruous in the sagittal plane and to avoid this, the patellar cartilage is thicker and does not follow the contour of the subchondral bone, in addition to being quite permeable and elastic; therefore, your contact area increases, decreasing the pressure. The patellar cartilage is the thickest in the body and therefore can withstand high imposed loads, but biomechanical changes can generate changes, causing pain and/or wear of the cartilage.

Due to the incongruence and the ability to move in relation to the femur, the contact on the patella changes with knee flexion and extension and the contraction force of the quadriceps. One of the causes of pain and wear is the increased pressure between the patella and the femur, which should be avoided, especially by those who already have the injury. In knee flexion, the quadriceps performs a force facing upwards and the patella tendon supports the quadriceps force in the opposite direction, making a resultant in the posterior direction, causing, then, the increased compression between the patella and the femur (HAUPENTHAL, 2006).

Studies by Eisenhart (2004) show that patellofemoral contact occurs from 30 degrees of knee flexion and increases as the angle increases.

According to Kisner (2005), excessive lateral displacement of the patella characterizes it as patella alta and may occur due to the imbalance between the lateral and medial compartments of the quadriceps.

Patella alta, or rather structural patellar tilt, results from shortening of the lateral retinaculum as an adaptive process, which abnormally increases the load on the lateral facet, reducing and distorting the weight on the medial and distal facet (FELD, 2000).

For Felkerson (2000) there is normally a wide distribution of contact along the distal patella at 30 degrees of knee flexion. It is evident that an alteration, even if small, in the patellofemoral alignment, can create load peaks in the articular cartilage that, eventually, can promote pathological alterations in the joint, such as chondromalacia. Muscular imbalance of the medial and lateral quadriceps compartments represents the highest incidence of chondromalacia cases (KISNER, 2005).

As previously reported, the vastus lateralis is the strongest muscle of the quadriceps. If it is actively working in the knee extensor mechanism, pulling the patella upwards and laterally and if there is no equal counter force from the medial compartment, there will be a tendency to excessive lateral displacement, causing increased tension and shortening of the vastus lateralis and iliotibial band, hypotonia and weakness of the vastus medialis. In this case, the vastus medialis should be strengthened to pull the patella medially and avoid medial retinacular stretch and lateral retinacular tension (GABRIEL, 2001).

The musculature of the human body is composed of different types of fibers given the scientific name of type I fibers, intermediate fibers II, type IIa fibers, and IIb fibers. These fibers are stimulated in different ways so to speak the fibers of type I are known as red fibers or slow oxidative these fibers they present a dark red color thus showing the highest concentration of hemoglobin, they are of slow contraction, therefore they present more resistance to fatigue. Type II fibers are the fast twitch fibers or white fibers, these fibers she has as main factor the rapid contraction by atp pathways anaerobically, where there is a greater lactic fermentation, and phosphocreatine predominating glycolytic pathway, they activate explosively thus differentiating it from type I because the same can not provide such a level of contraction. (GUYTON; HALL, 2011)

The same authors also mention that type IIa fibers are intermediate fibers where there are higher levels of anaerobic fibers, but also have a large amount of mitochondria and oxidative enzymes resulting in resistance capacity. Type IIb fibers are practically anaerobic fibers, as they are destroyed from myoglobin thus becoming white fibers, with minimal mitochondria thus metabolizing only glucose, beta-oxidation and Krebs cycle do not occur, causing the great accumulation of blood lactate and H + post exercise.

According to Zachary et al. (2013) the physiology of each type of muscle fiber we can have an idea about what the RFS will stimulate, according to his page total hypertrophy, described that the RFS in the practice of resistance exercise with weight occurs a large accumulation of lactate, stimulation of GH, fatigue of type I fibers, greater recruitment of type II fibers, release of nitric oxide synthase (NOS-1), inhibition of myostatin, release of IGF-1, phosphorylation activation of the Akt / mTOR pathway, all of these with a single objective muscle growth hypertrophy. Thus proving to be a beneficial method for gaining strength and muscle mass.

According to Guyton and Hall (2011) for muscle contraction to occur, there is a physiological form of this muscle contraction, before the act of muscle contractiona occurs there is a neural motor command where it takes such a command that part of the brain by motor neuron, neurons that carry the nervous command to specific muscles, by neuron axons, where it travels through these neuron axons and reaching the muscle cell where it takes the muscle contraction command.

The author cited above, says that during the command of the nerve impulse for contraction, the motor neuron carries information through a nerve impulse to the end of the motor neuron where it is called the motor plate that is attached to the muscle fibers, the nerve ending it releases a chemical substance called acetylcholine where it is responsible for conducting the act of the motor command to the muscle fiber (muscle cell), where chemical elements such as sodium are released in this way occurring the action potential, thus making the inversion of electrical charges and this inversion in the muscle cells will occur muscle contraction.

The neuron in it has an electrochemical electrical charge, has a positive electrical charge and internally there is a negative charge, there are channels in these neurons where sodium is taken into this neuron and potassium out where there is an inversion of polarity, occurring the nerve impulse through the sodium and potassium pump, it is transmitted from point to point of the axon until it reaches the muscle fiber thus transmitting the nerve conduction. Through this nerve impulse the motor plate releases acetylcholine in contact with the sarcoplasmic reticulum that is in the muscle fibers and perpetuates itself throughout the muscle fiber thus opening another channel releasing the calcium so that muscle contraction occurs.

According to Guyton and Hall (2011) The muscle is composed of sarcomere which is a structural unit of the muscle delimits the Z lines, actinin main protein of thin filaments and myosin which is the main protein thick filaments, to reach the nerve conduction along with troponin, tropomyosin, atp and ions câlcios these are the components of muscle contraction and relaxation. The myosin it is composed of two intertwined tails and two heads they are responsible for contracting or pulling the actin, in the sarcomere the several myosin filaments joined between them, which are positioned in different ways in the contraction the myosin fibers bind to the actin filaments thus promoting muscle contraction, thus occurring in several stages for contraction and relaxation to occur.

The same author also states that to promote this contraction there must be an action potential as already mentioned above, so it will cause the calcium to be released from the sarcoplasmic reticulum to the sarcoplasm of the muscle cell and it will bind to tropin there will be an effect on troponin and tropomyosin, this effect is basically opening for the myosin head to bind to actin, in the myosin head there is an ATP receptor where it and it is hydrolyzed thus providing energy to the myosin head, and this displacement causes the fibers to contract, for the relaxation of the fibers to occur it is necessary that there is ATP once again in the myosin head occurring relaxation, and this causes the muscle to perform another contraction. And so that a new contraction does not occur in the sarcoplasmic reticulum, where an energy pump will occur capturing the calcium into the sarcoplasmic reticulum, this calcium coming out of troponin it blocks the myosin bond and contraction does not occur, for the contraction to occur again a new action potential is necessary, and this is an extremely fast dynamic process for contraction and relaxation to occur.

3.1 Energy sources

There are energy sources that are necessary for the practice of exercise. There are two types of energy sources, aerobic and anaerobic, aerobic energy sources the priorities of this type of exercise have as a wedge to extract energy from this substrate oxygen, already in anaerobic exercises does not have oxygen as an energy source, but phosphocreatine that has great power in a short time, phosphocreatine is a short-term energy, when this energy source falls, due to its short period of time as an energy source, glucose takes over as an energy source for the realization of exercise in a strong way thus providing a significant amount. Where without the presence of oxygen it begins to produce lactate, where without the presence of oxygen glucose it is transformed into lactate acid and this lactate acid and transformed into lactate, and consequently occurs a muscular acidosis where the muscle is with the PH but low, where it is observed in the practice of anaerobic exercise muscle burning. (SANTOS, 2004).

The aforementioned author also says that these energy sources are consumed in the daily life of the human being as proteins, carbohydrates and fats. Where these substances produce energy needed to maintain body functions both for the body at rest and in exercise practice, these substances in the practice of exercises are used in different ways depending on the intensity of the exercise as previously cited aerobic and anaerobic exercises. In anaerobic exercise is performed over a long period of time where it is low intensity, the muscles need long-lasting stimuli, thus recruiting type I fibers oxidative fibers, this exercise has oxygen as its energy source. Already in anaerobic its main source of energy as already mentioned above is phosphocreatine and glucose. For energy to occur, glucose is broken down into ATP (adenosine triphosphate), so energy is propagated in the muscle through the breakdown of ATP.

3.2 Hypertrophy and strength

According to Vinay et al. (2005) Hypertrophy is defined by hyper (large) trophy (volume), for a hypertrophic response is necessary chemical or physical stimuli, there are the main mediators to increase muscle volume are TGF-Д IGF- 1, alpha-adrenergic agonist, endothelin 1, angiotesin II, mechanical stretch and some steroid hormones and peptides.

Muscle damage is undoubtedly one of the main factors for muscle hypertrophy to occur, muscle hypertrophy also occurs due to several other factors, which are subdivided into intrinsic factors (intensification of eccentric contraction of the musculature occurring a higher level of tissue microlesion, hormonal and enzymatic factors, such as increased GH, IGF-I, Testosterone, Insulin and Myostatin, satellite cells) all these factors will be stimulated and obtained with the practice of resistance training with weight (TRP). (GUYTON; HALL, 2011)

The microlesôes occurred in the myofibrils, take the body in a physiological way to act so that tissue healing occurs, this process increases the synthesis of contractile proteins thus leading to the regenerative process of muscle fibers, in this way the synthesis increases the cross section giving it a greater volume thus leading to muscle hypertrophy. In this way it can be observed that the muscle cell by its healing process of the damage was increased in volume.

Muscle strength is closely related to the greater recruitment of muscle fibers, the greater activation of motor units, as we saw above in the physiology of contraction and types of muscle fibers, in the physiology of muscle contraction it was seen that for contraction to occur a stimulus is needed, this stimulus comes in the central nervous system. And also as noted above in the types of muscle fibers there are some types of fibers and different specificities type I fibers, type II fibers, type IIa fibers and type IIb fibers, was seen each one definitively. (NELIO, 2003)

The same author also states that in strength training today is much demand for young people, adults and the elderly, because it is not only for aesthetic means, but also as quality of life, prevention and rehabilitation. For strength training to be successful it is necessary to associate it with TRP (resistance training with weight), in this way it will have good results. An important relationship of muscle strength is its tension generated during exercise the greater the tension (overload) the greater the recruitment of fibers and the greater the muscle strength, the type of fibers that are activated in strength training is the type II fibers, type IIa and type IIb are fibers that are related to the powers not only of strength, but also energetic and speed of contraction. There are three types of muscle action concentric, eccentric and isometric, the length of the musculature changes according to each action in the concentric decreases, in the eccentric increases and in the isometric does not change, so the concentric and eccentric considered the main ones for the gain of muscle strength with TRP.

CHAPTER 4 - METHODOLOGICAL APPROACH

4.1 Research design

This is a case series study with a quantitative methodological approach.

According to Gil (2011) the case study is punctuated by the application of deep, determined and exhaustive, of few or some objects, so that your knowledge is evident, understandable and detailed. This type of study is widely used to explore situations which are not clearly defined, to describe the context of the situation investigated, as well as to explain causes of certain episodes or occurrences in situations that do not allow experiments.

The aforementioned author describes that the exploratory research have as crucial points to develop, clarify and modify concepts and ideas through a more precise problematization or hypotheses for possible further studies, involving bibliographical research, documentary, interviews and case study, where the final product becomes a more clarified problem. The descriptive type of research aims to describe the characteristics of a given population or phenomenon, however, there are researches that, although defined as descriptive according to their objectives, end up serving more to provide a new view of the problem, which brings them closer to exploratory research.

The research was carried out at G mais Academia, located at Av: Tancredo Neves, 353, Mandacaru, in the period of April and May 2017. The sample consisted of a woman who was selected according to the inclusion criteria of the research which was: physically healthy woman, aged between 18 and 60 years, height of 1.50 to 1.90m and who presents patellar chondropathy in at least one of the knees. The exclusion criteria adopted were: women who used anabolic steroids, had systemic arterial hypertension, cardiopulmonary problems and muscle injuries.

The present study was carried out in the bodybuilding room of G plus Academy, where some equipment was used such as: (extensor chair, bar and washers, flexor table, abductor chair, standing or sitting flexor and sentadilha or machine for calves). A table of exercises for the respective muscle groups was protocoled: hamstrings, quadriceps, iliotibial tract and triceps sural.

The 1RM test according to the protocol of Baechle and Earle, (2010), was performed in the extensor chair and flexor table (Vitally), it is necessary that the exercises are always performed with correct form and technique to ensure the accuracy of the measurement. Body perimetry was performed on lower limbs and a pre- and post-intervention assessment. The pain identification test was also performed where the numerical pain scale will be applied (Appendix B).

The warm-up was performed on a treadmill (Movement, LX 160) for 5 minutes, the pressure applied to the thighs was made with aneroid sphygmomanometer (PREMIUM), and also the specific warm-up using 50% of the load in the execution of the movement that works the lower limb specifically thighs. The research participant was instructed not to practice any other type of counter-resistance training during the research.

The exercises were performed, according to the intervention protocol (Appendix C), in the extensor chair, free squat with weight, flexor table, flexor standing unilateral or sitting bilateral and sit-up. The exercises were performed in isokinetic contraction, until muscle fatigue, doing three sets of each exercise and resting from one exercise to the other from 3 to 5mim without vascular restriction. All exercises that were performed with vascular restriction, had a rest between one series and another of 40 to 50sec with vascular restriction, vascular restriction was only removed after the end of one type of exercise to be able to move on to the other.

The intervention lasted six weeks with two weekly sections, the exercise was performed with vascular restriction, with an intensity of 20% of 1RM and the sphygmomammometer was placed near the inguinal fold of the thighs (MMII).

The present project was appreciated by the Collegiate of the Physiotherapy Course and submitted to the evaluation of the Ethics and Research Committee was approved with CAE of n°66479317.8.0000.5178 by the CEP of the Faculty of Medical Sciences of Paraiba, through the sending of the project to Plataforma Brasil. Emphasizing that for the realization of the proposed study will be obeyed all the criteria established by Resolution 466/12 of the National Health Council (CNS) on ethics in research with human beings.

The participation of the individual was voluntary, as well as clarifying all doubts to the participants through the information elaborated in a Free and Informed Consent Form (ICF) (Appendix A) that explained about the research in a clear way, showing objectives, benefits and functioning of the study, in addition to referring through this, verbal clarifications and the guarantee of confidentiality of the data collected, in addition to being informed about their freedom to withdraw their consent at any stage of the study.

It is considered that in all research involving human beings there are risks, as well as in anyone who practices training or rehabilitation there may be risks. According to Allan and Borba (2013), some articles show that there are risks for people who will perform training with vascular occlusion, such as DVT (deep vein thrombosis) that can cause a pulmonary embolism if not resolved, due to total vascular restriction for a long time. Where it can also cause an increase in blood pressure during the execution of training, decreased cardiac output, decreased cerebral flow, where evidence shows that there is a greater risk of thrombosis, congestive heart failure and hematological diseases. In this study, so that no physical and emotional damage occurs, the research will be carried out in a preventive manner for such risks, where it will work in the pressure safety margin that studies recommend that are safe for individuals, which is from lOOmmhg to 200mmhg, in case some of these risks presented above occur, the participant will be directed to the scope of specialty of the risk suffered thus having all the assistance of the researchers. The same (volunteer) will have all the information about the risks that may suffer, and if it occurs what should be done to improve it in the TCLE (Appendix A). The academic researcher in charge will be trained in the applicability of the technique, thus eliminating the risk.

According to Allan and Borba (2013), the benefits analyzed in articles of different methodological designs showed that the vast majority had the same benefit of increasing muscle cross-section and increasing muscle strength, using only 20% to 50% of 1RM. Despite the different training executions and pressure values, it was seen that both in trained and untrained individuals and individuals in hospital beds had good results, both in increasing muscle volume and strength, as well as in preserving factors such as diapensia and muscle hypotrophy.

With the increase in muscle strength that involves the knee, there is a gain of stability in this joint, thus consequently leading to improvement of pain and better functionality. For physiotherapy it is a very good method for rehabilitation of patients with chondropathy, because most patients who do not present any contraindication, can use this method of training supervised by a trained professional who knows the subject, taking into account the use of small kilograms and training loads, preventing other complications, gaining muscle mass and strength to improve physical condition, functionality and pain reduction.

The data analysis of this research was quantitative, where the data were analyzed through descriptive statistics (mean, percentage), using the Windows Excel program, thus being presented in the form of tables and graphs.

4.2 Results and discussion

The research sample consisted of a female volunteer with chondropathy, the age range given by the research was 18 to 60 years old, sociodemographic data were evaluated according to the evaluation form, cardiac problems, osteomioarticular problems, hypertension, pain scale, as well as the perimetry of the MMII and 1RM test according to the Baechle and Earle protocol, (2010), the volunteer presented grade II chondropathy and a pain scale in 8. The present research was carried out in 12, twice weekly.

In the pre-intervention the 1RM test was performed, evaluating the volunteer in all the machines mentioned above as extensor chair, flexor table, flexor chair, squat, abductor chair, calf on the machine, the test was performed with the patient / volunteer performing a maximum repetition with high kilages, not being able to perform the mechanical movement of the machine was given 5 minutes of decay for the next realization of the same movement, as well as the other exercises thus performing in all machines and the following data were collected table 1 1RM test.

Table 1: 1RM test assessing muscle strength pre-intervention

1RM TEST Pre-intervention	
Extension chair	50kg
Flex table	45kg
Flexor chair	42kg
Abductor chair	55kg
Squatting	30kg
Calf machine	40kg

Source: SILVA; PAIVA, 2017

As was also performed the perimetry test of MMII and triceps sural evaluating as follows thighs supra patellar of 5cm, 7cm, 10cm, 14cm, 21cm, and triceps sural of 7cm and 14cm of calcaneus towards the popliteal force evaluating with measuring tape, the following data were collected table 2.

Table 2: evaluation of perimetry of lower limbs and triceps sural assessing muscle trophism.

Perimetry Pre-intervention			
Left Thigh	Right Thigh	Tricepssural left	Right triceps sural
5 cm 52,5	5cm 52	7cm 40,5	7cm 40,5
7cm 53	7cm 56	14cm 33	14cm 36,5
10cm 55,5	10cm 58		
14cm 55	14cm 63		
21cm 64, 5	21cm 71		

Source: SILVA; PAIVA, 2017

After intervention, new 1RM test data were collected, thus demonstrating a good evolution of the patient / volunteer, where she showed significant strength gains to those evaluated in the pre-intervention, the 1RM test was performed in the same way as the pre-intervention, always respecting the rest time of 5min between one execution and another, the following results were collected table 3.

Table 3: 1RM evaluation showing the evolution in strength gain.

1RM TEST	
Post intervention	
Extension chair	70kg
Flex table	60kg
Flexor chair	67kg
Abductor chair	75kg
Squatting	45kg
Calf machine	55kg

Source: SILVA; PAIVA, 2017

According to the study by Takarada, et al. 2000, where he shows us that training with vascular occlusion really there is a significant gain in muscle strength the present study carried out in a weight room with the patient / volunteer who had grade II chondropathy, also had a good evolution in the gain of muscle strength thus proving what was said in the study of the author mentioned above.

In the perimetry test where we evaluated the muscular trophism in circumference of the MMII and triceps sural, did not observe a good gain in muscle mass, believed that due to the short intervention time only 12 sections, 6 weeks twice weekly.

Table 4: evaluation of perimetry of lower limbs and triceps sural assessing muscle trophism.

Perimetry Post intervention			
Post intervention			
Left Thigh	Right Thigh	Tricepssural left	Right triceps sural
5 cm 53,5	5cm 53,5	7cm 41,5	7 cm 42
7cm 54,3	7cm 58,5	14cm 34,5	14cm 38
10cm 56,8	10cm 59		

| 14cm 56 | 14cm 63,8 | |
| 21cm 65,6 | 21cm 72,4 | |

Source: SILVA; PAIVA, 2017

It was not possible to observe a good gain in muscle trophism believing that only 12 sessions of training were performed, thus comparing to the study of FLECK, S. J. et al. 2017 which shows that muscle trophism through training can only be observed after approximately three months of training, thus proving the lack of muscle mass gain even using the vascular occlusion method in training.

In the pain scale presented by the patient/volunteer where she reported an intensity of 8, so collected in the initial evaluation where she presented joint crepitations in the left knee, where she sought to do an imaging examination and was proven chondropathy grade II, was performed all the intervention and then reassessed post intervention where the volunteer presented great evolution in joint pain reduction table 5.

Table 5: pain scale pre and post intervention

Pain scale	
Pre-intervention	Post intervention
Pain scale 8	Pain scale 2

Source: SILVA; PAIVA, 2017

After the consultations, she reported a good evolution, believing that with the gain of muscle strength, thus generating a good joint stabilization, she could present this good evolution according to Nakajima et al. 2006 where this method is not only used in gyms as a form of training, but also in hospitals and rehabilitation clinics in Japan, thus demonstrating its great effectiveness not only in the form of training to gain strength and hypertrophy but also using these objectives to gain joint stabilization as was performed in the present study thus proving a good evolution in the pain condition of the patient / volunteer.

FINAL CONSIDERATIONS

According to some authors the training using blood vascular restriction which is a training using a specific sphygmomanometer or the normal Premium brand, involving the MMSS or MMII thus decreasing the blood flow of the site, and practicing resistance training, has a strong evolution in muscle mass gain and strength using only 20% to 50% of 1RM, thus showing that to have a gain in muscle mass and strength is not necessary to work with high kilograms or train with 70% to 85% of 1RM, as shown in other methods of resistance training (LOENNEKE et al., 2012).

Another very important factor in this training method is the significant increase in GH (human growth hormone) in blood plasma compared to other training methods. The accumulation of metabolites consequently increases the concentration of GH, this increase was verified in other studies after exercise, a study carried out with young people using vascular occlusion proved that after exercise there is a large increase and accumulation of GH in the blood plasma, where also the greater electrical activity in muscle activity thus recruiting more muscle fibers in the execution of the exercise, the authors also concluded that the gradual increase in lactate in the blood plasma during exercise combined also with hypoxia leading to greater recruitment of motor units. Thus recruiting larger amounts of motor units coming to the conclusion that a significant gain not only of strength, but also of muscle hypertrophy. (TAKARADA et al., 2000)

Chondropathy refers to diseased cartilage. This condition usually causes pain in the front of the knee and clicking, especially when the person squats, runs, gets up from a chair or goes up and down stairs. The more specific term for this condition is patellofemoral syndrome. The highest incidences in women in relation to the Q angle, which is the relationship between the knee hip between the knee patella and lateral part of the antero superior iliac hip, the misalignment of this angle leads the knees to be inward in valgus in this way the patella is more lateralized promoting greater wear of the cartilage during movement, very common in women because of having the hip be wider due to genetic characteristics due to pregnancy the relationship and also little strength in the knee stabilizing muscles such as the iliotibial tract, quadriceps (BRUKNER et al. 2006).

Thus seeing the great importance of this training in the face of the need to work with low kilograms in patients with osteomioatic lesions such as patellar chondropathy where we must work with low kilograms and achieve a good result, it was seen the great need to work with training with vascular occlusion to obtain an improvement in stabilization with gain of muscle strength and hypertrophy and most importantly the reduction of the painful symptomatology generated by patellar chondropathy.

In the first care the volunteer reported a muscle burning when performing the exercises, thus proving what was reported in Takarada et al, (2000) thus showing the presence of lactate in the musculature, thus promoting the increase of micro muscle injury. As well as having performed the exercises until muscle exhaustion the same presented strong fatigue in MMII as well as muscle pain post training because of this report were given 48hrs for the next training section thus working according to the physiology of muscle recovery as written in the book of Guyton and Hall, 2011.

The research volunteer showed a significant strength gain where after the 12 sections a new test was performed as shown in table 3, muscle hypertrophy did not have much significance table 4, because according to FLECK, S. J. et al. 2017 only the increase in cross-section of the musculature is presented a good gain in muscle mass after approximately three months, as already in the pain scale presented by the patient in the pre-intervention had a good evolution after the intervention table 5.

REFERENCES

ABE, T. et al. Blood flow restriction pressure recommendations: The hormesis hypothesis. **Medical Hypothesis**, v 82, p 623-626, 2014.

BRUKNER, Peter D. et al. 5. Recent advances in sports medicine. **Medical Journal of Australia**, v. 184, n. 4, p. 188, 2006.

FLECK, Steven J.; KRAEMER, William J. **Fundamentals of muscle strength training**. Artmed Publishing House, 2017.

GUYTON, A. C.; HALL, J. E. Treatise on Medical Physiology. 12th Ed. Rio de Janeiro: Elsevier Ltda. 2011.

LOENNEKE, J. P.; THIEBAUD, R. S.; ABE, T. Does blood flow restriction result in skeletal muscle damage? A critical review of available evidence. **Scandinavian journal of medicine & science in sports**, v. 24, n. 6, p. e415-422, 2014.

LOENNEKE, J. P. et al. Blood flow restriction pressure recommendations: the hormesis hypothesis. **Medical hypotheses**, v. 82, n. 5, p. 623-626, 2014.

LOENNEKE, J. P. et al. Blood flow restriction: how does it work? **Frontiers in physiology**, v. 3, 2012.

LOENNEKE, Jeremy et al. Blood flow restriction: an evidence based progressive model (Review). **Acta Physiologica Hungarica**, v. 99, n. 3, p. 235-250, 2012.
KARABULUT et al. Effects of high-intensity resistance training and low-intensity resistance
NAKAJIMA T, KURANO M, IIDA H, TAKANO H, OONUMA H, MORITA T, ET AL.
Use and safety of KAATSU training: results of a national survey. **International Journal of**

KAATSU Training Research.v.2, n. 1, p. 5-13, 2006.

PATRICK, A. W. et al. Analysis of the hemodynamic and vascular repercussions of kaatsu training. **ConScientiae Saude**, v.12 n. 2, p.305-312, 2013.

POPE, Zachary K.; WILLARDSON, Jeffrey M.; SCHOENFELD, Brad J. Exercise and blood flow restriction. **The Journal of Strength & Conditioning Research**, v. 27, n. 10, p. 29142926, 2013.

POTON, R.; POLITO, M. D.; Cardiovascular Responses during Resisted Exercise with Blood Flow Restriction. **Rev Bras Cardiol**, v. 27, n. 2, p. 104-110, 2014.

LENZI S. **Google analytics**. Available at: http://www.treinomestre.com.br/conheca-mais-about-the-kaatsu-training-method-japones-for-hypertrophy/, accessed October 25, 2016.

SANTOS, P. J. M. **Fisiologia do musculo esquelético**. Faculty of Physical Education of the University of Porto, v. 1, 2004.

TAKARADA Y, NAKAMURA Y, ARUGA S, ONDA T, MIYAZAKI S, ISHII N. Rapid increase in plasma growth hormone after low-intensity resistance exercise with vascular occlusion.J Appl Physiol, 88: 61-65, 2000.
TAKARADA Y, TAKAZAWA H, SATO Y, TAKEBAYASHI S, TANAKA Y, ISHII N. Effects of resistance exercise combined with moderate vascular occlusion on muscular function in humans. **J Appl Physiol.** 88(6):2097-106, 2000.

WERNBOM, M.; AUGUSTSSON, J.; RAASTAD, T. Ischemic strength training: a low load alternative to heavy resistance exercise? **Scandinavian journal of medicine & science in sports**, v. 18, n. 4, p. 401-416, 2008.

ZACHARY K. POPE, JEFFREY M. Willardson, and Brand J. Schoenfeld. Exercise and Blood Flow Restriction 2013.

34

ZANARDI, CAROLINE C.; LIMA, CRISTINA M. A. M. physiotherapeutic intervention in patients with patellofemoral syndrome. **Health and environment: interdisciplinary magazine**, v. 1, n. 1, p. 163-172, 2012.

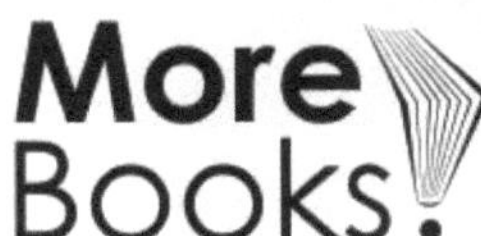

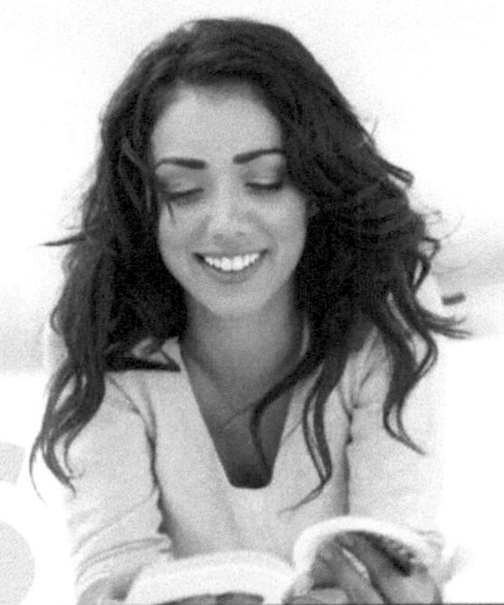

yes
I want morebooks!

Buy your books fast and straightforward online - at one of world's fastest growing online book stores! Environmentally sound due to Print-on-Demand technologies.

Buy your books online at
www.morebooks.shop

Kaufen Sie Ihre Bücher schnell und unkompliziert online – auf einer der am schnellsten wachsenden Buchhandelsplattformen weltweit! Dank Print-On-Demand umwelt- und ressourcenschonend produziert.

Bücher schneller online kaufen
www.morebooks.shop

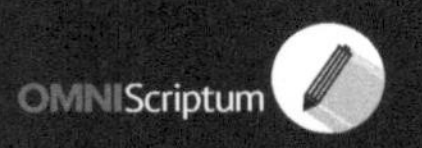

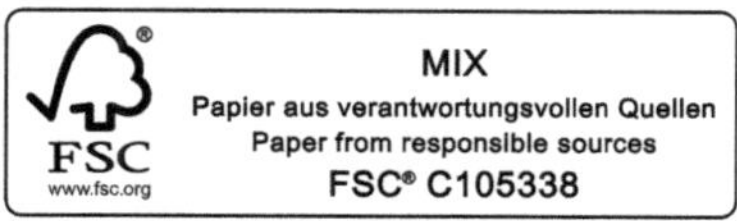

Printed by Books on Demand GmbH, Norderstedt / Germany